LEAN AND GREEN

AIR FRYER

COOKBOOK

Turbocharge your weight loss and health with these Seafood and Vegetable Air Fryer Recipes.

To my dear and passionate readers, seekers of novelty, taste, and better health. May you use these new recipes to reach your desired body weight goal and put new energy into being the change you want to see in this extraordinary life.

Contents

Introduction

The Lean and Green diet is a diet where the basic idea is to cut out junk food, eat only 'lean' meat, such as fish, poultry and vegetables and also drink a lot of green tea. This diet is said to be not only good for your health but also a good way to control weight. The diet claims to reduce your weight, as well as reducing the risk of gout and other diseases.

There have been many scientific studies on this diet over the years, which find that the diet can reduce excess weight, blood pressure and cholesterol levels.

The biggest advantage of this diet is that you do not need to count calories or anything like that. The diet is based on the concept that we only consume what we need in terms of calories – not more. The theory is that if you eat only a certain amount of food, your body will use its stored energy (fat) to convert the food into energy, so you will not gain weight.

Lean and Green is a concept which is very similar to the Atkins diet, but the main difference between Lean and Green and Atkins is that Lean and Green only allows you to eat foods which have a low glycemic index value.

The Glycemic Index (GI) is often used in scientific studies to determine how certain foods affect weight control. A food's GI value shows how much that food affects blood sugar levels. In the short term, this means that you can eat more of a low GI food than a high GI food. In the long term though, a diet high in low GI foods is healthier.

In the "Lean and green" diet, you are not allowed to eat any carbohydrates which have a GI value above 50. Also, you are not allowed to drink milk. This means that you can eat only fish, poultry and vegetables such as carrots and broccoli.

The main disadvantage of this diet is that it does not take into consideration your body type or physical constitution (i.e. whether you are ectomorphic or mesomorphic). The diet is good for anyone who wants to lose weight, but it is only a weight loss diet.

However, many people believe that this diet is more than just the best way to lose weight. The Lean and Green diet also aims to reduce the risk of several diseases and claims that it is a low-calorie diet. Although there are some studies suggesting that the diet reduces blood pressure and cholesterol levels, these claims have not been proven yet.

Lean and green diet has proven to be extremely helpful in controlling and maintaining weight. Still, when lean & green food merges with air frying, it can make this diet much easier for people to follow. Air frying food cuts the cooking time in half and makes the food more nutritious.

Air frying is an innovative heat cooking method that is gaining popularity in India. In practical terms, cooking is done without oil. Preparing food using methods like air frying along with lean and green foods, it can give better results.

With the advent of health-conscious people, more and more people are also turning into this diet to lose weight and remain healthy. Most people are already aware that the air fryer is a great and healthy way to prepare food, but it is not so popular to opt for.

The air fryer works by blasting a heating element and circulating heated air inside a rotating drum filled with the food that is being prepared.

This diet is commonly followed by people who are looking for a successful way to lose weight. The diet is different from all the other diets followed by people around the globe. This diet plan is a success story, a mind-boggling one.

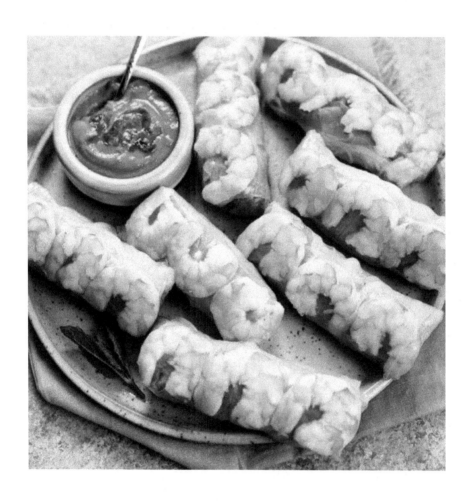

Seafood Recipes

1. Shrimp Spring Rolls

Difficulty: Average

Preparation Time: 9 minutes

Cooking Time: 25 minutes

Servings: 4

Ingredients

- Deveined raw shrimp: half cup chopped(peeled) (1 lean)

- Olive oil: 2 and 1/2 tbsp. (1/8 condiment)

- Matchstick carrots: 1 cup (1/2 green)

- Slices of red bell pepper: 1 cup (1/2 green)

- Red pepper: 1/4 teaspoon(crushed) (1/4 green)

- Shredded cabbage: 2 cups (1 green)

- Lime juice: 1 tablespoon (1/8 condiment)

- Sweet chili sauce: half cup (1/8 condiment)

- Fish sauce: 2 teaspoons (1/8 condiment)

- Eight spring roll(wrappers) (1 healthy fat)

Direction

1. In a skillet, add one and a half tbsp. of olive, until smoking lightly. Stir in bell pepper, cabbage, carrots, and cook for two minutes. Turn off the heat, take out in a dish and cool for five minutes.

2. In a bowl, add shrimp, lime juice, cabbage mixture, crushed red pepper, and fish sauce. Mix well

3. Lay spring roll wrappers on a plate. Add 1/4 cup of filling in the middle of each wrapper. Fold tightly with water. Brush the olive oil over folded rolls.

4. Put spring rolls in the air fryer basket and cook for 6 to 7 minutes at 390°F until light brown and crispy.

5. You may serve with sweet chili sauce.

Nutrition:

- 180 Calories

- 9g Fat

- 17g Protein

2. Air Fryer Scallops with Tomato Cream Sauce

Difficulty: Average

Preparation Time: 5 minutes

Cooking Time: 10 minutes

Servings: 2

Ingredients

- Sea scallops eight jumbo (4 lean)

- Tomato Paste: 1 tbsp. (1/4 condiment)

- Chopped fresh basil 1 tablespoon (1/2 green)

- 3/4 cup of low-fat Whipping Cream (1/2 healthy fat)

- Kosher salt half teaspoon (1/4 condiment)

- Ground Freshly black pepper half teaspoon (1/4 condiment)

- Minced garlic 1 teaspoon (1/4 condiment)

- Frozen Spinach, thawed half cup (1/2 green)

Direction

1. Take a seven-inch pan(heatproof) and add spinach in a single layer at the bottom

2. Rub olive oil on both sides of scallops, season with kosher salt and pepper.

3. on top of the spinach, place the seasoned scallops

4. Put the pan in the air fryer and cook for ten minutes at 350F, until scallops are cooked completely, and the internal temperature reaches 135F.

5. Serve immediately.

Nutrition:

- 259 Calories

- 19g Protein

- 13g Fat

3. Sriracha & Honey Tossed Calamari

Difficulty: Easy

Preparation Time: 9 minutes

Cooking Time: 20 minutes

Servings: 2

Ingredients

- Club soda: 1 cup (1/2 condiment)

- Sriracha: 1-2 Tbsp. (1/4 condiment)

- Calamari tubes: 2 cups (1 lean)

- Flour: 1 cup (1/2 healthy fat)

- Pinches of salt, freshly ground black pepper, red pepper flakes, and red pepper (1/4 condiment)

- Honey: 1/2 cup (1/2 healthy fat)

Direction

1. Cut the calamari tubes into rings. Submerge them with club soda. Let it rest for ten minutes.

2. In the meantime, in a bowl, add freshly ground black pepper, flour, red pepper, and kosher salt and mix well.

3. Drain the calamari and pat dry with a paper towel. Coat the calamari well in the flour mix and set aside.

4. Spray oil in the air fryer basket and put calamari in one single layer.

5. Cook at 375 for 11 minutes. Toss the rings twice while cooking. Meanwhile, to make sauce honey, red pepper flakes, and sriracha in a bowl, well.

6. Take calamari out from the basket, mix with sauce, cook for another two minutes more. Serve with salad green.

Nutrition

- 252 Calories

- 38g Fat

- 41g Protein

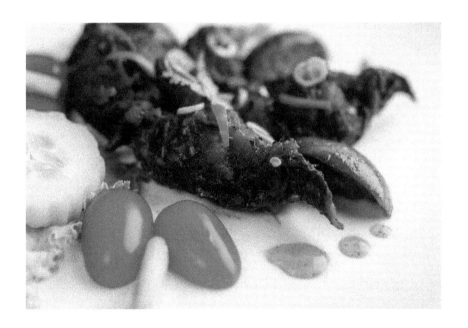

4. Air Fryer Southern Style Catfish with Green Beans

Difficulty: Average

Preparation Time: 8 minutes

Cooking Time: 23 minutes

Servings: 2

Ingredients

- Catfish fillets: 2 pieces (1 lean)

- Green beans: half cup, trimmed (1/2 green)

- Honey: 2 teaspoons (1/4 condiment)

- black pepper and salt, to taste (1/4 condiment)

- Crushed red pepper: half tsp. (1/2 green)

- Flour: 1/4 cup (1/4 condiment)

- One egg, lightly beaten (1/2 healthy fat)

- Dill pickle relish: 3/4 teaspoon (1/4 condiment)

- Apple cider vinegar: half tsp (1/4 condiment)

- 1/3 cup whole-wheat breadcrumbs (1/2 healthy fat)

- Mayonnaise: 2 tablespoons (1/4 condiment)

- Dill (1/2 green)

- Lemon wedges (1/4 condiment)

Direction

1. In a bowl, add green beans, spray them with cooking oil. Coat with crushed red pepper, 1/8 teaspoon of kosher salt, and half tsp. Of honey and cook in the air fryer at 400 F until soft and browned, for 12 minutes. Take out from fryer and cover with aluminum foil

2. In the meantime, coat catfish in flour. Then dip in egg to coat, then in breadcrumbs. Place fish in an air fryer basket and spray with cooking oil.

3. Cook for 8 minutes, at 400F.

4. Sprinkle with pepper and salt. In the meantime, mix vinegar, dill, relish, mayonnaise, and honey in a bowl. Serve the sauce with fish and green beans.

Nutrition:

- 243 Calories

- 18g fat

- 33g Protein

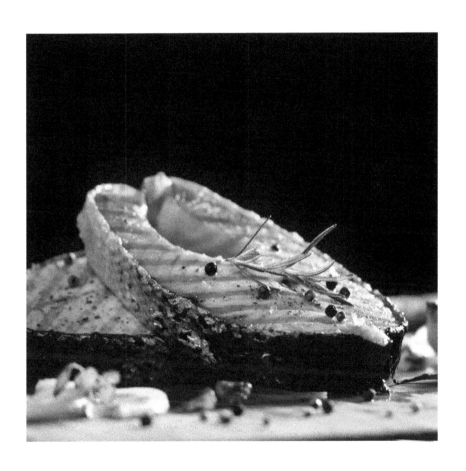

5. Roasted Salmon with Fennel Salad

Difficulty: Easy

Preparation Time: 14 minutes

Cooking Time: 9 minutes

Servings: 4

Ingredients

- Skinless and center-cut: 4 salmon fillets (2 lean)

- Lemon juice: 1 teaspoon(fresh) (1/8 condiment)

- Parsley: 2 teaspoons(chopped) (1/4 green)

- Salt: 1 teaspoon, divided (1/8 condiment)

- Olive oil: 2 tablespoons (1/8 condiment)

- Chopped thyme: 1 teaspoon (1/4 green)

- Fennel heads: 4 cups (thinly sliced) (1/4 green)

- One clove of minced garlic (1/8 condiment)

- Fresh dill: 2 tablespoons, chopped (1/4 green)

- Orange juice: 2 tablespoons(fresh) (1/2 healthy fat)

- Greek yogurt: 2/3 cup(reduced-fat) (1/2 healthy fat)

Direction

1. In a bowl, add half teaspoon of salt, parsley, and thyme, mix well. Rub oil over salmon, and sprinkle with thyme mixture.

2. Put salmon fillets in the air fryer basket, cook for ten minutes at 350°F.

3. In the meantime, mix garlic, fennel, orange juice, yogurt, half tsp. of salt, dill, lemon juice in a bowl.

4. Serve with fennel salad.

Nutrition:

- 364 Calories

- 30g Fat

- 38g Protein

6. Air Fryer Catfish with Cajun Seasoning

Difficulty: Easy

Preparation Time: 5 minutes

Cooking Time: 27 minutes

Servings: 4

Ingredients

- Cajun seasoning: 3 teaspoons (1/2 condiment)

- Cornmeal: 3/4 cup (1/2 healthy fat)

- 4 catfish fillets (2 lean)

Direction

1. In a zip lock bag, add Cajun seasoning and cornmeal

2. Wash and pat dry the catfish fillets. Add them to the zip lock bag.

3. Coat well the fillets with seasoning

4. Put catfish fillets in the air fryer and cook for 15 minutes at 390 F, turn fillets halfway through. To get a golden color on the fillets, cook for five more minutes.

5. Serve with lemon wedges and spicy tartar sauce.

Nutrition

- 324 Calories

- 14g Fat

- 26.3g Protein

7. Air Fryer Sushi Roll

Difficulty: Difficult

Preparation Time: 91 minutes

Cooking Time: 9 minutes

Servings: 3

Ingredients

For the Kale Salad

- Rice vinegar: half teaspoon (1/8 condiment)

- Chopped kale: one and a 1/2 cups (1/2 green)

- Garlic powder:1/8 teaspoon (1/8 condiment)

- Sesame seeds: 1 tablespoon (1/4 healthy fat)

- Toasted sesame oil: 3/4 teaspoon (1/8 condiment)

- Ground ginger: 1/4 teaspoon (1/8 condiment)

- Soy sauce: 3/4 teaspoon (1/8 condiment)

Sushi Rolls

- Half avocado - sliced (1/2 healthy fat)

- Cooked Sushi Rice - cooled (1 healthy fat)

- Whole wheat breadcrumbs: half cup (1/2 healthy fat)

- Sushi: 3 sheets (1 lean)

Direction

Make the Kale Salad

1. In a bowl, add vinegar, garlic powder, kale, soy sauce, sesame oil, and ground ginger. With your hands, mix with sesame seeds and set them aside.

Sushi Rolls

2. Lay a sheet of sushi on a flat surface. With damp fingertips, add a tablespoon of rice, and spread it on the sheet. Cover the sheet with rice, leaving half-inch space at one end.

3. Add kale salad with avocado slices. Roll up the sushi, use water if needed.

4. Add the breadcrumbs in a bowl. Coat the sushi roll with Sriracha Mayo, then in breadcrumbs.

5. Add the rolls to the air fryer. Cook for ten minutes at 390 F, shake the basket halfway through.

6. Take out from the fryer, and let them cool, then cut with a sharp knife.

7. Serve with soy sauce.

Nutrition:

- 369 Calories

- 13.9g Fat

- 26g Protein

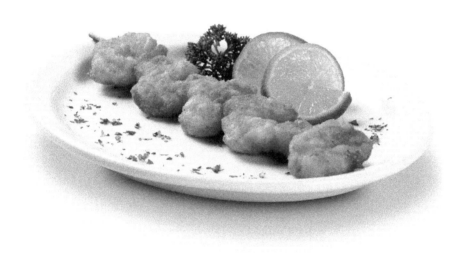

8. Air Fryer Garlic-Lime Shrimp Kebabs

Difficulty: Easy

Preparation Time: 5 minutes

Cooking Time: 19 minutes

Servings: 2

Ingredients

- 1 lime (1/4 condiment)

- Raw shrimp: 1 cup (1 lean)

- Salt: 1/8 teaspoon (1/4 condiment)

- 1 clove of garlic (1/4 condiment)

- Freshly ground black pepper (1/4 condiment)

Direction

1. In water, let wooden skewers soak for 20 minutes.

2. Let the Air fryer preheat to 350F.

24

3. In a bowl, mix shrimp, minced garlic, lime juice, kosher salt, and pepper

4. Add shrimp on skewers.

5. Place skewers in the air fryer, and cook for 8 minutes. Turn halfway over.

6. Top with cilantro and your favorite dip.

Nutrition:

- 76 Calories

- 13g Protein

- 9g fat

9. Fish Finger Sandwich

Difficulty: Average

Preparation Time: 10 minutes

Cooking Time: 9 minutes

Servings: 4

Ingredients

- Greek yogurt: 1 tbsp. (1/2 healthy fat)

- Cod fillets: 4, without skin (2 lean)

- Flour: 2 tbsp. (1/4 healthy fat)

- Whole-wheat breadcrumbs: 5 tbsp. (1/4 healthy fat)

- Kosher salt and pepper, to taste (1/4 condiment)

- Capers: 10–12 (1/2 healthy fat)

- Lemon juice (1/4 condiment)

Direction

1. Let the air fryer preheat.

2. Sprinkle kosher salt and pepper on the cod fillets, and coat in flour, then in breadcrumbs

3. Spray the fryer basket with oil. Put the cod fillets in the basket.

4. Cook for 15 minutes at 200 C.

5. In the meantime, blend with Greek yogurt, lemon juice, and capers until well combined.

6. On a bun, add cooked fish with pea puree. Add lettuce and tomato.

Nutrition:

- 240 Calories

- 12g Fat

- 20g Protein

10. Healthy Air Fryer Tuna Patties

Difficulty: Easy

Preparation Time: 15 minutes

Cooking Time: 11 minutes

Servings: 10

Ingredients

- Whole wheat breadcrumbs: half cup (1/4 healthy fat)

- Fresh tuna: 4 cups, diced (2 lean)

- Lemon zest (1/4 condiment)

- Lemon juice: 1 Tablespoon (1/4 condiment)

- 1 egg (1/4 healthy fat)

- Grated parmesan cheese: 3 Tablespoons (1/4 healthy fat)

- One chopped stalk celery (1 green)

- Garlic powder: half teaspoon (1/4 condiment)

- Dried herbs: half teaspoon (1/4 green)

- Salt to taste (1/8 condiment)

- Freshly ground black pepper (1/8 condiment)

Direction

1. In a bowl, add lemon zest, bread crumbs, salt, pepper, celery, eggs, dried herbs, lemon juice, garlic powder, parmesan cheese, and onion. Mix everything. Then add in tuna gently. Shape into patties. If the mixture is too loose, cool in the refrigerator.

2. Add air fryer baking paper in the air fryer basket. Spray the baking paper with cooking spray.

3. Spray the patties with oil.

4. Cook for ten minutes at 360°F. Turn the patties halfway over.

5. Serve with lemon slices and microgreens.

Nutrition:

- 214 Calories

- 15g Fat

- 22g Protein

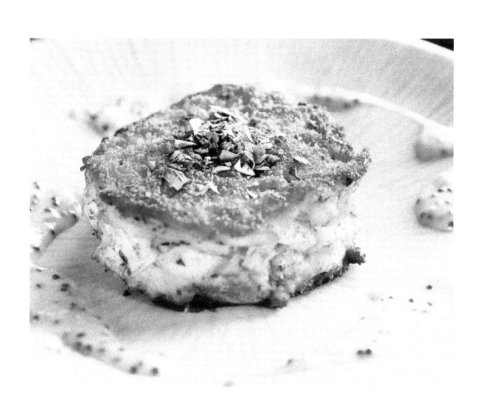

11. Crab Cakes

Difficulty: Average

Preparation Time: 14 minutes

Cooking Time: 19 minutes

Servings: 6

Ingredients

- Crab meat: 4 cups (2 lean)

- 2 eggs (1 healthy fat)

- Whole wheat bread crumbs: ¼ cup (1/2 healthy fat)

- Mayonnaise: 2 tablespoons (1/2 healthy fat)

- Worcestershire sauce: 1 teaspoon (1/4 condiment)

- Old Bay seasoning: 1 and ½ teaspoon (1/4 condiment)

- Dijon mustard: 1 teaspoon (1/4 condiment)

- Black pepper to taste (1/4 condiment)

- Green onion: ¼ cup, chopped (1/4 green)

Direction

1. In a bowl, add Dijon mustard, Old Bay, eggs, Worcestershire, and mayonnaise mix it well. Then add in the chopped green onion and mix.

2. Fold in the crab meat to mayonnaise mix. Then add breadcrumbs, not to over mix.

3. Chill the mix in the refrigerator for at least 60 minutes. Then shape into patties.

4. Let the air-fryer preheat to 350F. Cook for 10 minutes. Flip the patties halfway through.

5. Serve with lemon wedges.

Nutrition:

- 218 Calories

- 13g Fat

- 17g Protein

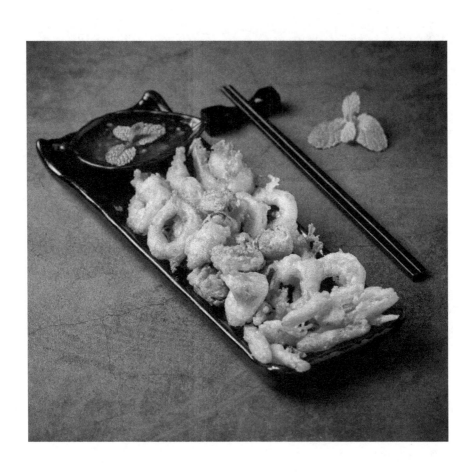

12. Breaded Air Fried Shrimp with Bang-Bang Sauce

Difficulty: Difficult

Preparation Time: 9 minutes

Cooking Time: 22 minutes

Servings: 4

Ingredients

- Whole wheat bread crumbs: 3/4 cup (1/2 healthy fat)

- Raw shrimp: 4 cups, deveined, peeled (2 lean)

- Flour: half cup (1/8 condiment)

- Paprika: 1 tsp (1/8 condiment)

- Chicken Seasoning, to taste (1/8 condiment)

- 2 tbsp. of one egg white (1/2 healthy fat)

- Kosher salt and pepper to taste (1/8 condiment)

Bang-Bang Sauce

- Sweet chili sauce: 1/4 cup (1/8 condiment)

- Plain Greek yogurt: 1/3 cup (1/3 healthy fat)

- Sriracha: 2 tbsp. (1/8 condiment)

Direction

1. Let the Air Fryer preheat to 400 degrees.

2. Add the seasonings to shrimp and coat well.

3. In three separate bowls, add flour, bread crumbs, and egg whites.

4. First coat the shrimp in flour, dab lightly in egg whites, then in the bread crumbs.

5. With cooking oil, spray the shrimp.

6. Place the shrimps in an air fryer, cook for four minutes, turn the shrimp over, and cook for another four minutes. Serve with micro green and bang-bang sauce.

Bang-Bang Sauce

7. Incorporate all the ingredients and serve.

Nutrition:

- 229 calories

- 10g fat

- 22g protein

13. Air Fryer Crispy Fish Sandwich

Difficulty: Easy

Preparation Time: 11 minutes

Cooking Time: 12 minutes

Servings: 2

Ingredients

- Cod :2 fillets (1 lean)

- All-purpose flour: 2 tablespoons (1/4 condiment)

- Pepper: 1/4 teaspoon (1/8 condiment)

- Lemon juice: 1 tablespoon (1/4 condiment)

- Salt: 1/4 teaspoon (1/8 condiment)

- Garlic powder: half teaspoon (1/8 condiment)

- One egg (1/2 healthy fat)

- Mayo: half tablespoon (1/4 healthy fat)

- Whole wheat bread crumbs: half cup (1/2 healthy fat)

Direction

1. In a bowl, add salt, flour, pepper, and garlic powder.

2. In a separate bowl, add lemon juice, mayo, and egg.

3. In another bowl, add the breadcrumbs.

4. Coat the fish in flour, then in egg, then in breadcrumbs.

5. With cooking oil, spray the basket and put the fish in the basket. Also, spray the fish with cooking oil.

6. Cook at 400 F for ten minutes. This fish is soft, be careful if you flip.

Nutrition:

- 218 Calories

- 12g Fat

- 22g Protein

14. Easy Shrimp Egg Rolls

Difficulty: Average

Preparation Time: 24 minutes

Cooking Time: 19 minutes

Servings: 6

Ingredients

- 2-3 cloves of minced garlic (1/2 condiment)

- 12-14 egg roll wrappers (1 healthy fat)

- Raw shrimp (roughly chopped): 4 cups, peeled and deveined (2 lean)

- Coleslaw mix: 3 cups (1 healthy fat)

- Sesame oil: 1 and 1/2 teaspoons (1/8 condiment)

- Soy sauce: 1 tablespoon (1/4 condiment)

- Fish sauce: 1 teaspoon (1/8 condiment)

- Salt, pepper to taste (1/8 condiment)

- Grated ginger: half tsp. (1/8 condiment)

- Two green onions chopped (1 green)

- Water: one cup (1/4 condiment)

Direction

1. In a skillet, add shrimp with garlic, kosher salt, and pepper, spray with cooking oil and sauté until shrimp is pink. Put off the heat and set it aside.

2. In a bowl, add coleslaw mix, cooked shrimp, green onions, fish sauce, soy sauce, sesame oil, and ginger. Mix well.

3. Add two tbsp. Of filling, in each wrapper, seal tightly with water.

4. With cooking oil, spray the air fryer basket. Situate egg rolls in a single layer in the basket. Spray with cooking oil.

5. Cook for 7 minutes at 400 degrees. Flip the rolls, then cook for five minutes more.

6. Serve with micro green salad.

Nutrition:

- 228 calories

- 11g fat

- 20g protein

15. Easy Shrimp PO' Boy

Difficulty: Easy

Preparation Time: 19 minutes

Cooking Time: 9 minutes

Servings: 4

Ingredients

- Iceberg lettuce: 2 cups shredded (1 green)

- Shrimp:4 cups, deveined (2 lean)

- Buttermilk: 1/4 cup (1/4 healthy fat)

- Fish Fry Coating: 1/2 cup (1/4 condiment)

- Creole Seasoning: 1 teaspoon (1/8 condiment)

- Eight slices of tomato (1/2 green)

Remoulade Sauce

- Creole Seasoning: half tsp. (1/8 condiment)

- Mayo: half cup(reduced-fat) (1/2 healthy fat)

- Half lemon's juice (1/8 condiment)

- Dijon mustard: 1 tsp (1/8 condiment)

- Worcestershire: 1 tsp (1/8 condiment)

- Minced garlic: one tsp. (1/8 condiment)

- One green onion chopped (1/4 condiment)

- Hot sauce: one tsp

Direction

Remoulade Sauce

1. Mix all ingredients in a bowl. Chill in Refrigerator.

Shrimp

2. In a zip lock bag, add buttermilk and Creole seasoning with shrimp and mix well, marinate for half an hour.

3. With cooking oil, spray the air fryer basket. Place the shrimp in the air fryer basket.

4. Spray the shrimp with olive oil.

5. Cook at 400 F for five minutes. Flip the shrimps over, and cook for extra five minutes.

6. Add the remoulade sauce on whole-wheat bread. Then add tomato slices and lettuce on top, then the shrimp. Enjoy

Nutrition:

- 247 Calories

- 19.3g fat

- 24.7g protein

16. Quick & Easy Air Fryer Salmon

Difficulty: Easy

Preparation Time: 6 minutes

Cooking Time: 13 minutes

Servings: 4

Ingredients

- Lemon pepper seasoning: 2 teaspoons (1/4 condiment)

- Salmon: 4 cups (2 lean)

- Olive oil: one tablespoon (1/4 condiment)

- Seafood seasoning: 2 teaspoons (1/4 condiment)

- Half lemon's juice (1/4 condiment)

- Garlic powder:1 teaspoon (1/8 condiment)

- Kosher salt to taste (1/8 condiment)

Direction

1. In a bowl, add one tbsp. of olive oil and half lemon juice.

2. Pour this mixture over salmon and rub. Leave the skin on salmon. It will come off when cooked.

3. Rub the salmon with kosher salt and spices.

4. Put parchment paper in the air fryer basket. Put the salmon in the air fryer.

5. Cook at 360 F for ten minutes. Cook until inner salmon temperature reaches 140 F.

6. Let the salmon rest five minutes before serving.

7. Serve with salad greens and lemon wedges.

Nutrition:

- 132 Calories

- 7.4g fat

- 22g protein

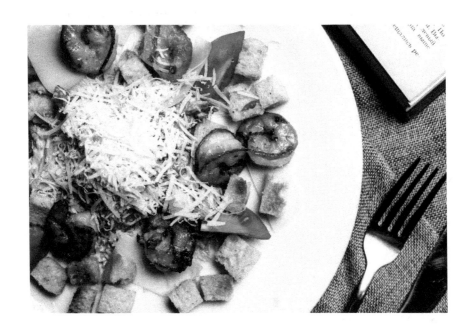

17. Air Fryer Parmesan Shrimp

Difficulty: Average

Preparation Time: 6 minutes

Cooking Time: 12 minutes

Servings: 4

Ingredients

- Olive oil: 2 tablespoons (1/2 condiment)

- Jumbo cooked shrimp: 8 cups, peeled, deveined (4 lean)

- Parmesan cheese: 2/3 cup(grated) (1/2 healthy fat)

- Pepper: 1 teaspoon (1/4 condiment)

- 4 cloves of minced garlic (1/2 condiment)

- Oregano: 1/2 teaspoon (1/4 green)

- Basil: 1 teaspoon (1/4 green)

- Lemon wedges (1/2 condiment)

Direction

1. Mix parmesan cheese, onion powder, oregano, olive oil, garlic, basil, and pepper in a bowl. Coat the shrimp in this mixture.

2. Spray oil on the air fryer basket, put shrimp in it.

3. Cook for ten minutes, at 350 F, or until browned.

4. Drizzle the lemon on shrimps before serving with a microgreen salad.

Nutrition:

- 198 Calories

- 13g Fat

- 12.7g Protein

18. Air Fryer Lemon Garlic Shrimp

Difficulty: Average

Preparation Time: 6 minutes

Cooking Time: 12 minutes

Servings: 2

Ingredients

- Olive oil: 1 Tbsp. (1/4 condiment)

- Small shrimp: 4 cups, peeled, tails removed (2 lean)

- One lemon juice and zest (1/4 condiment)

- Parsley: 1/4 cup sliced (1/4 green)

- Red pepper flakes(crushed): 1 pinch (1/4 condiment)

- Four cloves of grated garlic (1/8 condiment)

- Sea salt: 1/4 teaspoon (1/8 condiment)

Direction

1. Let air fryer heat to 400F

2. Mix olive oil, lemon zest, red pepper flakes, shrimp, kosher salt, and garlic in a bowl and coat the shrimp well.

3. Place shrimps in the air fryer basket, coat with oil spray.

4. Cook at 400 F for 8 minutes. Toss the shrimp halfway through

5. Serve with lemon slices and parsley.

Nutrition:

- 140 Calories

- 18g Fat

- 20g Protein

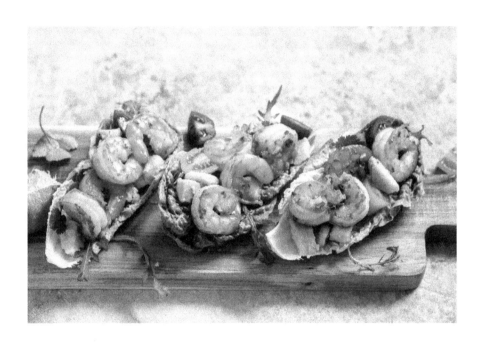

19. Air Fryer Shrimp Tacos

Difficulty: Average

Preparation Time: 16 minutes

Cooking Time: 16 minutes

Servings: 4

Ingredients

- Flour tortillas: 12 (2 healthy fat)

- Avocado sliced: 1 cup (1/4 healthy fat)

- Chipotle chili powder: 1 tsp (1/8 condiment)

- Raw jumbo shrimp: 24 pieces, deveined, peeled, without tail (4 lean)

- Smoked paprika: 1/2 tsp (1/8 condiment)

- Salt: 1/4 tsp (1/8 condiment)

- Olive oil: 1 tbsp. (1/8 condiment)

- Green salsa: ½ cup (1/4 healthy fat)

- Light brown sugar: 1 and 1/2 tsp (1/8 condiment)

- Garlic powder: 1/2 tsp (1/8 condiment)

- Low-fat sour cream: 1/2 cup (1/4 healthy fat)

Direction

1. Let the oven preheat to 400 F and spray the air fryer basket with oil spray.

2. In a bowl, mix chipotle chili powder, salt, brown sugar, smoked paprika, and garlic powder, mix well

3. Pat dry the shrimp, put shrimp in zip lock bag and add the seasonings and toss to coat well

4. Place shrimp in air fryer basket in one even layer, cook for four minutes and flip them overcook for four minutes more

5. For the sauce, mix sour cream and green salsa.

6. Put shrimp in a tortilla, top with sauce, shrimp, sliced avocado serves with lime wedges.

Nutrition:

- 228 Calories

- 18g Fat

- 20g Protein

20. Air Fryer Lemon Pepper Shrimp

Difficulty: Average

Preparation Time: 6 minutes

Cooking Time: 11 minutes

Servings: 2

Ingredients

- Raw shrimp: 1 and 1/2 cup peeled, deveined (1 lean)

- Olive oil: 1/2 tablespoon (1/4 condiment)

- Garlic powder: ¼ tsp (1/8 condiment)

- Lemon pepper: 1 tsp (1/4 condiment)

- Paprika: ¼ tsp (1/8 condiment)

- Juice of one lemon (1/4 condiment)

Direction

1. Let the air fryer preheat to 400 F

2. In a bowl, mix lemon pepper, olive oil, paprika, garlic powder, and lemon juice. Mix well. Add shrimps and coat well

3. Add shrimps in the air fryer, cook for 6 or 8 minutes and top with lemon slices and serve

Nutrition:

- 237 Calories

- 6g Fat

- 36g Protein

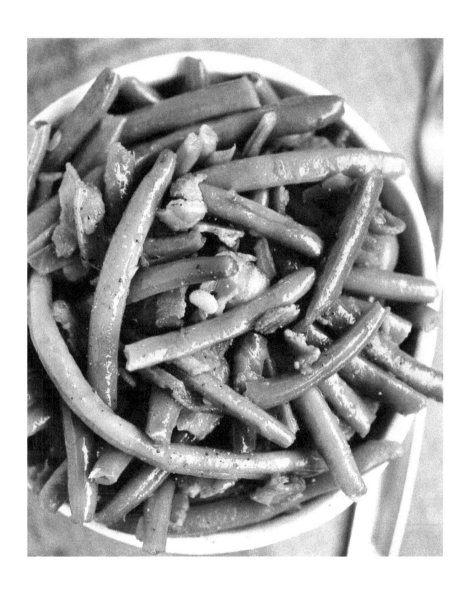

Vegetable Recipes

21. Healthy & Tasty Green Beans

Difficulty: Easy

Preparation Time: 10 minutes

Cooking Time: 10 minutes

Servings: 2

Ingredients:

- 2 cups green beans (1/2 green)

- 1/8 tsp ground allspice (1/8 condiment)

- 1/4 tsp ground cinnamon (1/8 condiment)

- 1/2 tsp dried oregano (1/4 green)

- 2 tbsp olive oil (1/8 condiment)

- 1/4 tsp ground coriander (1/8 condiment)

- 1/4 tsp ground cumin (1/8 condiment)

- 1/8 tsp cayenne pepper (1/8 condiment)

- 1/2 tsp salt (1/8 condiment)

Directions:

1. Add all ingredients into the bowl and toss well.

2. Add green beans into the air fryer basket and cook at 370 F for 10 minutes. Shake basket halfway through

3. Serve and enjoy.

Nutrition

- 158 Calories

- 14g Fat

- 2.1g Protein

22. Cheesy Brussels Sprouts

Difficulty: Easy

Preparation Time: 10 minutes

Cooking Time: 12 minutes

Servings: 4

Ingredients:

- 1 lb. Brussels sprouts, cut stems and halved (1/2 green)

- 1/4 cup parmesan cheese (1/2 healthy fat)

- 1 tbsp olive oil (1/4 condiment)

- 1/4 tsp garlic powder (1/4 condiment)

- Pepper (1/8 condiment)

- Salt (1/8 condiment)

Directions:

1. Preheat the air fryer to 350 F.

2. Toss Brussels sprouts, oil, garlic powder, pepper, and salt into the bowl.

3. Situate Brussels sprouts into the air fryer basket and cook for 12 minutes.

4. Top with cheese and serve.

Nutrition

- 132 Calories

- 7g Fat

- 7g Protein

23. Garlic Cauliflower Florets

Difficulty: Easy

Preparation Time: 10 minutes

Cooking Time: 20 minutes

Servings: 4

Ingredients:

- 4 cups cauliflower florets (1/2 green)

- 1/2 tsp cumin powder (1/8 condiment)

- 1/2 tsp coriander powder (1/8 condiment)

- 5 garlic cloves, chopped (1/8 condiment)

- 4 tablespoons olive oil (1/8 condiment)

- 1/2 tsp salt (1/8 condiment)

Directions:

1. Add all ingredients into the bowl and toss well.

2. Add cauliflower florets into the air fryer basket and cook at 400 F for 20 minutes. Shake halfway through.

3. Serve and enjoy.

Nutrition

- 153 Calories

- 14g Fat

- 2.3g Protein

24. Delicious Ratatouille

Difficulty: Difficult

Preparation Time: 10 minutes

Cooking Time: 15 minutes

Servings: 6

Ingredients:

- 1 eggplant, diced (1/2 green)

- 3 garlic cloves, chopped (1/4 condiment)

- 1 onion, diced (1/4 condiment)

- 3 tomatoes, diced (1/2 healthy fat)

- 2 bell peppers, diced (1/2 green)

- 1 tbsp vinegar (1/4 condiment)

- 1 1/2 tbsp olive oil (1/4 condiment)

- 2 tbsp herb de Provence (1/2 green)

- Pepper (1/8 condiment)

- Salt (1/8 condiment)

Directions:

1. Preheat the air fryer to 400 F.

2. Add all ingredients into the bowl and toss well.

3. Add vegetable mixture into the air fryer basket and cook for 15 minutes. Stir halfway through.

4. Serve and enjoy.

Nutrition

- 83 Calories

- 4g Fat

- 2g Protein

25. Simple Green Beans

Difficulty: Easy

Preparation Time: 10 minutes

Cooking Time: 10 minutes

Servings: 4

Ingredients:

- 2 cups green beans (1 green)

- 1 tsp olive oil (1/2 condiment)

- Pepper (1/4 condiment)

- Salt (1/4 condiment)

Directions:

1. In a bowl, toss green beans with oil. Season with pepper and salt.

2. Transfer green beans into the air fryer basket and cook at 390 F for 10 minutes.

3. Serve and enjoy.

Nutrition

- 27 Calories

- 1.2g Fat

- 1g Protein

26. Air Fryer Tofu

Difficulty: Easy

Preparation Time: 10 minutes

Cooking Time: 15 minutes

Servings: 4

Ingredients:

- 15 oz extra firm tofu, cut into bite-sized pieces (1 healthy fat)

- 1 tbsp olive oil (1/4 condiment)

- 2 tbsp soy sauce (1/4 condiment)

- 1 garlic clove, minced (1/4 condiment)

- Pepper (1/8 condiment)

- Salt (1/8 condiment)

Directions:

1. Add tofu, garlic, oil, soy sauce, pepper, and salt in a bowl and toss well. Set aside for 15 minutes.

2. Add tofu pieces into the air fryer basket and cook at 370 F for 15 minutes.

3. Serve and enjoy.

Nutrition

- 115 Calories

- 8g Fat

- 9.8g Protein

27. Healthy Zucchini Patties

Difficulty: Easy

Preparation Time: 10 minutes

Cooking Time: 30 minutes

Servings: 6

Ingredients:

- 1 cup zucchini, shredded and squeeze out all liquid (1/2 green)

- 1 egg, lightly beaten (1/4 healthy fat)

- 1/4 tsp red pepper flakes (1/4 condiment)

- 1/4 cup parmesan cheese, grated (1/4 healthy fat)

- 1/2 tbsp Dijon mustard (1/4 condiment)

- 1/2 tbsp mayonnaise (1/4 healthy fat)

- 1/2 cup breadcrumbs (1/2 healthy fat)

- Pepper (1/8 condiment)

- Salt (1/8 condiment)

Directions:

1. Mix all ingredients into the bowl until well combined.

2. Make patties from mixture and place them into the basket and cook at 375 F for 15 minutes.

3. Turn patties and cook for 15 minutes more.

4. Serve and enjoy.

Nutrition

- 80 Calories

- 3g Fat

- 4g Protein

28. Healthy Asparagus Spears

Difficulty: Easy

Preparation Time: 10 minutes

Cooking Time: 15 minutes

Servings: 4

Ingredients:

- 35 asparagus spears, cut the ends (2 green)

- 1/2 tsp garlic powder (1/4 condiment)

- 1 tbsp olive oil (1/4 condiment)

- Pepper (1/8 condiment)

- Salt (1/8 condiment)

- ¼ tsp. onion powder (1/4 condiment)

Directions:

1. Add asparagus into the large bowl. Drizzle with oil.

2. Sprinkle with onion powder, garlic powder, pepper, and salt. Toss well.

3. Arrange asparagus into the air fryer basket and cook at 375 F for 15 minutes.

4. Serve and enjoy.

Nutrition

- 75 Calories

- 4g Fat

- 4g Protein

29. Spicy Brussels Sprouts

Difficulty: Easy

Preparation Time: 10 minutes

Cooking Time: 14 minutes

Servings: 2

Ingredients:

- 1/2 lb. Brussels sprouts, trimmed and halved (1 lean)

- 1/2 tsp chili powder (1/4 condiment)

- 1/4 tsp cayenne (1/4 condiment)

- 1/2 tbsp olive oil (1/4 condiment)

- 1/4 tsp smoked paprika (1/4 condiment)

Directions:

1. Mix all ingredients into the large bowl and toss well.

2. Add Brussels sprouts into the air fryer basket and cook at 370 F for 14 minutes.

3. Serve and enjoy.

Nutrition

- 82 Calories

- 4g Fat

- 4g Protein

30. Cheese Broccoli Fritters

Difficulty: Average

Preparation Time: 10 minutes

Cooking Time: 30 minutes

Servings: 4

Ingredients:

- 2 eggs, lightly beaten (1/2 healthy fat)

- 3 cups broccoli florets, cook & mashed (1 lean)

- 2 cups cheddar cheese (1/2 healthy fat)

- 1/4 cup almond flour (1/4 condiment)

- 2 garlic cloves, minced (1/4 condiment)

- Pepper (1/4 condiment)

- Salt (1/4 condiment)

Directions:

1. Mix all ingredients into the bowl.

2. Make patties from mixture and place them into the basket and cook at 350 F for 15 minutes.

3. Turn patties and cook for 15 minutes more.

4. Serve and enjoy.

Nutrition

- 285 Calories

- 21g Fat

- 18g Protein

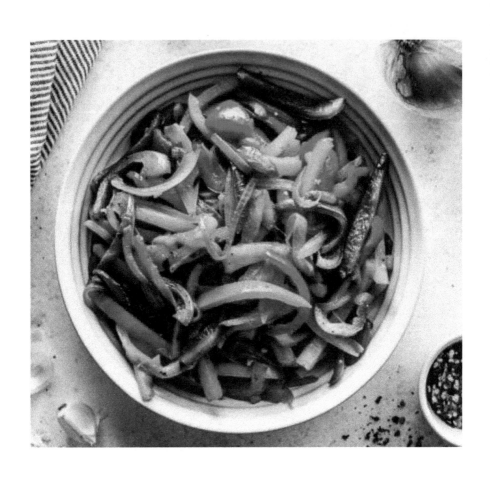

31. Air Fryer Bell Peppers

Difficulty: Easy

Preparation Time: 10 minutes

Cooking Time: 8 minutes

Servings: 3

Ingredients:

- ¼ tsp. onion powder (1/4 condiment)

- 3 cups bell peppers, cut into pieces (1 green)

- 1 tsp olive oil (1/2 condiment)

- 1/4 tsp garlic powder (1/4 condiment)

Directions:

1. Mix all ingredients into the large bowl and toss well.

2. Transfer bell peppers into the air fryer basket and cook at 360 F for 8 minutes. Stir halfway through.

3. Serve and enjoy.

Nutrition

- 52 Calories

- 2g Fat

- 1.2g Protein

32. Air Fried Tasty Eggplant

Difficulty: Easy

Preparation Time: 10 minutes

Cooking Time: 12 minutes

Servings: 2

Ingredients:

- 1 eggplant, cut into cubes (1 green)

- 1/4 tsp oregano (1/4 green)

- 1 tbsp olive oil (1/2 condiment)

- 1/2 tsp garlic powder (1/4 condiment)

- 1/4 tsp chili powder (1/4 condiment)

Directions:

1. Incorporate all ingredients into the huge bowl and toss well.

2. Transfer eggplant into the air fryer basket and cook at 390 F for 12 minutes. Stir halfway through.

3. Serve and enjoy.

Nutrition

- 120 Calories

- 7g Fat

- 2g Protein

33. Asian Green Beans

Difficulty: Average

Preparation Time: 10 minutes

Cooking Time: 10 minutes

Servings: 2

Ingredients:

- 8 oz green beans (1 green)

- 1 tbsp tamari (1/2 condiment)

- 1 tsp sesame oil (1/2 condiment)

Direction

1. Mix all ingredients into the big bowl and toss well.

2. Add green beans into the air fryer basket and cook at 400 F for 10 minutes.

3. Serve and enjoy.

Nutrition

- 60 Calories

- 2g Fat

- 3g Protein

34. Spicy Asian Brussels Sprouts

Difficulty: Average

Preparation Time: 10 minutes

Cooking Time: 15 minutes

Servings: 4

Ingredients:

- 1 lb. Brussels sprouts, cut in half (1 green)

- 1 tbsp gochujang (1/2 condiment)

- 1 1/2 tbsp olive oil (1/4 condiment)

- 1/2 tsp salt (1/4 condiment)

Directions:

1. In a bowl, mix olive oil, gochujang, and salt.

2. Add Brussels sprouts into the bowl and toss until well coated.

3. Add Brussels sprouts into the air fryer basket and cook at 360 F for 15 minutes.

4. Serve and enjoy.

Nutrition

- 94 Calories

- 5g Fat

- 4g Protein

35. Healthy Mushrooms

Difficulty: Easy

Preparation Time: 10 minutes

Cooking Time: 12 minutes

Servings: 2

Ingredients:

- 8 oz mushrooms, clean and cut into quarters (2 healthy fats)

- 1 tbsp fresh parsley, chopped (1/2 green)

- 1 tsp soy sauce (1/4 condiment)

- 1/2 tsp garlic powder (1/4 condiment)

- 1 tbsp olive oil (1/4 condiment)

- Pepper (1/8 condiment)

- Salt (1/8 condiment)

Directions:

1. Add mushrooms and remaining ingredients into the bowl and toss well.

2. Add mushrooms into the air fryer basket and cook at 380 F for 12 minutes. Stir halfway through.

3. Serve and enjoy.

Nutrition

- 90 Calories

- 7g Fat

- 4g Protein

36. Cheese Stuff Peppers

Difficulty: Average

Preparation Time: 10 minutes

Cooking Time: 8 minutes

Servings: 4

Ingredients:

- 10 jalapeno peppers, halved, remove seeds and stem (4 lean)

- 1/2 cup cheddar cheese (1/4 healthy fat)

- 1/2 cup Monterey jack cheese, shredded (1/4 healthy fat)

- 8 oz cream cheese, softened (1/2 healthy fat)

Directions:

1. In a bowl, mix together Monterey jack cheese and cream cheese.

2. Stuff cheese mixture into jalapeno halved.

3. Place jalapeno pepper into the air fryer basket and cook at 370 F for 8 minutes.

4. Serve and enjoy.

Nutrition

- 365 Calories

- 33g Fat

- 13.2g Protein

37. Cheesy Broccoli Cauliflower

Difficulty: Easy

Preparation Time: 10 minutes

Cooking Time: 20 minutes

Servings: 6

Ingredients:

- 4 cups cauliflower florets (1 green)

- 4 cups broccoli florets (1 green)

- 2/3 cup parmesan cheese, shredded (1 healthy fat)

- 5 garlic cloves, minced (1/2 condiment)

- 1/3 cup olive oil (1/4 condiment)

- Pepper (1/8 condiment)

- Salt (1/8 condiment)

Directions:

1. Add half cheese, broccoli, cauliflower, garlic, oil, pepper, and salt into the bowl and toss well.

2. Add broccoli and cauliflower to the air fryer basket and cook at 370 F for 20 minutes.

3. Add remaining cheese. Toss well.

4. Serve and enjoy.

Nutrition

- 165 Calories

- 13.6g Fat

- 6.4g Protein

38. Air Fryer Broccoli & Brussels Sprouts

Difficulty: Average

Preparation Time: 10 minutes

Cooking Time: 30 minutes

Servings: 6

Ingredients:

- 1 lb. Brussels sprouts, cut ends (1 green)

- 1 lb. broccoli, cut into florets (1 green)

- 1 tsp paprika (1/4 condiment)

- 1 tsp garlic powder (1/4 condiment)

- 1/2 tsp pepper (1/4 condiment)

- 3 tbsp olive oil (1 healthy fat)

- 3/4 tsp salt (1/4 condiment)

Directions:

1. Add all ingredients into the bowl and toss well.

2. Add vegetable mixture into the air fryer basket and cook at 370 F for 30 minutes.

3. Serve and enjoy.

Nutrition

- 125 Calories

- 7.6g Fat

- 5g Protein

39. Spicy Asparagus Spears

Difficulty: Easy

Preparation Time: 10 minutes

Cooking Time: 15 minutes

Servings: 4

Ingredients:

- 35 asparagus spears, cut the ends (2 green)

- 1/2 tsp chili powder (1/4 condiment)

- 1/4 tsp paprika (1/4 condiment)

- 1 tbsp olive oil (1/4 condiment)

- Pepper (1/8 condiment)

- Salt (1/8 condiment)

Directions:

1. Add asparagus into the large bowl. Drizzle with oil.

2. Sprinkle with paprika, chili powder, pepper, and salt. Toss well.

3. Add asparagus into the air fryer basket and cook at 400 F for 15 minutes.

4. Serve and enjoy.

Nutrition

- 75 Calories

- 3.8g Fat

- 4.7g Protein

40. Stuffed Mushrooms

Difficulty: Average

Preparation Time: 10 minutes

Cooking Time: 8 minutes

Servings: 16

Ingredients:

- 16 mushrooms, clean and chop stems (3 healthy fats)

- 2 garlic cloves, minced (1/2 condiment)

- 1/2 tsp chili powder (1/4 condiment)

- 1/4 cup cheddar cheese, shredded (1/2 healthy fat)

- 2 oz crab meat, chopped (1 lean)

- 8 oz cream cheese, softened (1/2 healthy fat)

- 1/4 tsp pepper (1/4 condiment)

Directions:

1. In a bowl, mix cheese, mushroom stems, chili powder, pepper, crabmeat, cream cheese, and garlic until well combined.

2. Stuff mushrooms with cheese mixture and place them into the air fryer basket and cook at 370 F for 8 minutes.

3. Serve and enjoy.

Nutrition

- 65 Calories

- 5.3g Fat

- 2.6g Protein

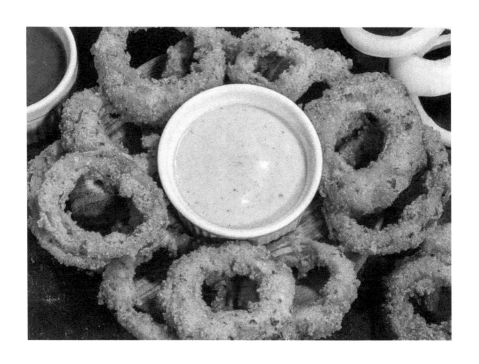

41. Almond Flour Battered 'n Crisped Onion Rings

Difficulty: Average

Preparation Time: 10 minutes

Cooking Time: 15 minutes

Servings: 3

Ingredients:

- ½ cup almond flour (1/4 healthy fat)

- ¾ cup coconut milk (1/4 healthy fat)

- 1 big white onion, sliced into rings (1 green)

- 1 egg, beaten (1/4 healthy fat)

- 1 tablespoon baking powder (1/4 condiment)

- 1 tablespoon smoked paprika (1/4 condiment)

- Salt and pepper to taste (1/8 condiment)

Directions:

1. Preheat the air fryer for 5 minutes.

2. In a mixing bowl, mix the almond flour, baking powder, smoked paprika, salt and pepper.

3. In another bowl, combine the eggs and coconut milk.

4. Soak the onion slices into the egg mixture.

5. Dredge the onion slices in the almond flour mixture.

6. Place in the air fryer basket.

7. Close and cook for 15 minutes at 3250F.

8. Halfway through the cooking time, shake the fryer basket for even cooking.

Nutrition:

- 217 Calories

- 5.3g Protein

- 18g Fat

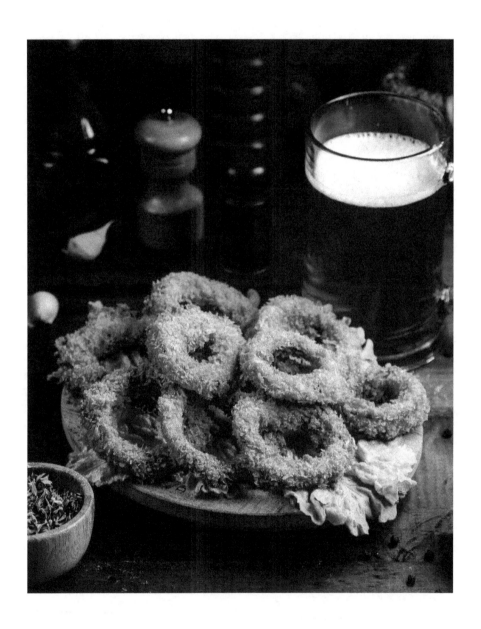

42. Tomato Bites with Creamy Parmesan Sauce

Difficulty: Easy

Preparation Time: 7 minutes

Cooking Time: 13 minutes

Servings: 4

Ingredients:

For the Sauce:

- 1/2 cup Parmigiano-Reggiano cheese, grated (1/4 healthy fat)

- 4 tablespoons pecans, chopped (1/2 healthy fat)

- 1 teaspoon garlic puree (1/8 condiment)

- 1/2 teaspoon fine sea salt (1/8 condiment)

- 1/3 cup extra-virgin olive oil (1/8 condiment)

For the Tomato Bites:

- 2 large-sized Roma tomatoes, cut into thin slices and pat them dry (1 green)

- 8 ounces Halloumi cheese, cut into thin slices (1 healthy fat)

- 1 teaspoon dried basil (1/2 green)

- 1/4 teaspoon red pepper flakes, crushed (1/8 condiment)

- 1/8 teaspoon sea salt (1/8 condiment)

Directions:

1. Start by preheating your Air Fryer to 385 degrees F.

2. Make the sauce by mixing all ingredients, except the extra-virgin olive oil, in your food processor.

3. While the machine is running, slowly and gradually pour in the olive oil; puree until everything is well - blended.

4. Now, spread 1 teaspoon of the sauce over the top of each tomato slice. Place a slice of Halloumi cheese on each tomato slice. Top with onion slices. Sprinkle with basil, red pepper, and sea salt.

5. Transfer the assembled bites to the Air Fryer. Spray with non-stick cooking spray and cook for about 13 minutes.

6. Arrange these bites on a nice serving platter, garnish with the remaining sauce, and serve at room temperature. Bon appétit!

Nutrition:

- 428 Calories

- 38g Fat

- 18g Protein

43. Simple Green Beans with Butter

Difficulty: Easy

Preparation Time: 2 minutes

Cooking Time: 10 minutes

Servings: 4

Ingredients:

- 3/4-pound green beans, cleaned

- 1 tablespoon balsamic vinegar

- 1/4 teaspoon kosher salt

- 1/2 teaspoon mixed peppercorns, freshly cracked

- 1 tablespoon butter

- 2 tablespoons toasted sesame seeds to serve

Directions:

1. Set your Air Fryer to cook at 390 degrees F.

2. Mix the green beans with all of the above ingredients, apart from the sesame seeds. Set the timer for 10 minutes.

3. Meanwhile, toast the sesame seeds in a small-sized nonstick skillet; make sure to stir continuously.

4. Serve sautéed green beans on a nice serving platter sprinkled with toasted sesame seeds. Bon appétit!

Nutrition:

- 73 Calories

- 3g Fat

- 1.6g Protein

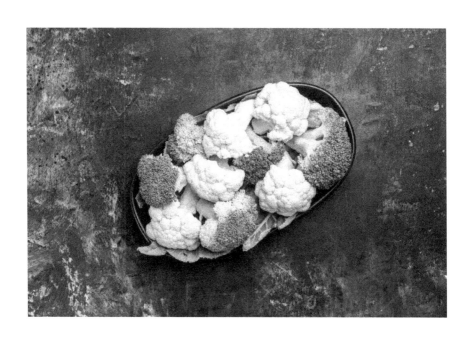

44. Creamy Cauliflower and Broccoli

Difficulty: Average

Preparation Time: 4 minutes

Cooking Time: 16 minutes

Servings: 6

Ingredients:

- 1-pound cauliflower florets (1 green)

- 1-pound broccoli florets (1 green)

- 2 ½ tablespoons sesame oil (1/2 condiment)

- 1/2 teaspoon smoked cayenne pepper (1/4 condiment)

- 3/4 teaspoon sea salt flakes (1/4 condiment)

- 1 tablespoon lemon zest, grated (1/4 condiment)

- 1/2 cup Colby cheese, shredded (1/2 healthy fat)

Directions:

1. Prepare the cauliflower and broccoli using your favorite steaming method. Then, drain them well; add the sesame oil, cayenne pepper, and salt flakes.

2. Air-fry at 390 degrees F for approximately 16 minutes; make sure to check the vegetables halfway through the cooking time.

3. Afterward, stir in the lemon zest and Colby cheese; toss to coat well and serve immediately!

Nutrition:

- 133 Calories

- 9g Fat

- 6g Protein

45. Mediterranean-Style Eggs with Spinach

Difficulty: Easy

Preparation Time: 3 minutes

Cooking Time: 12 minutes

Servings: 2

Ingredients:

- 2 tablespoons olive oil, melted (1/4 condiment)

- 4 eggs, whisked (1 healthy fat)

- 5 ounces' fresh spinach, chopped (1 green)

- 1 medium-sized tomato, chopped (1 green)

- 1 teaspoon fresh lemon juice (1/4 condiment)

- 1/2 teaspoon coarse salt (1/8 condiment)

- 1/2 teaspoon ground black pepper (1/8 condiment)

- 1/2 cup of fresh basil, roughly chopped (1/4 green)

Directions:

1. Add the olive oil to an Air Fryer baking pan. Make sure to tilt the pan to spread the oil evenly.

2. Simply combine the remaining ingredients, except for the basil leaves; whisk well until everything is well incorporated.

3. Cook in the preheated oven for 8 to 12 minutes at 280 degrees F. Garnish with fresh basil leaves. Serve.

Nutrition:

- 274 Calories

- 23g Fat

- 14g Protein

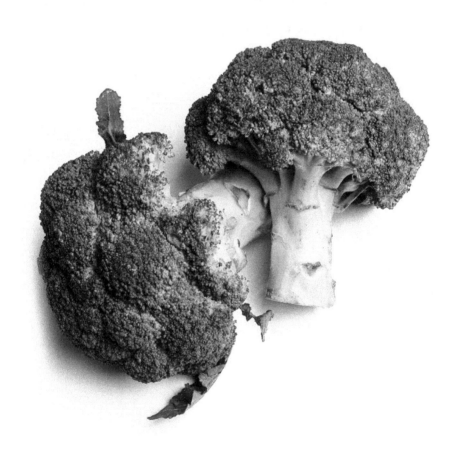

46. Spicy Zesty Broccoli with Tomato Sauce

Difficulty: Average

Preparation Time: 5 minutes

Cooking Time: 15 minutes

Servings: 6

Ingredients:

For the Broccoli Bites:

- 1 medium-sized head broccoli, broken into florets (1 green)

- 1/2 teaspoon lemon zest, freshly grated (1/4 condiment)

- 1/3 teaspoon fine sea salt (1/8 condiment)

- 1/2 teaspoon hot paprika (1/8 condiment)

- 1 teaspoon shallot powder (1/8 condiment)

- 1 teaspoon porcini powder (1/8 condiment)

- 1/2 teaspoon granulated garlic (1/8 condiment)

- 1/3 teaspoon celery seeds (1/4 healthy fat)

- 1 ½ tablespoons olive oil (1/8 condiment)

For the Hot Sauce:

- 1/2 cup tomato sauce (1/2 healthy fat)

- 1 tablespoon balsamic vinegar (1/8 condiment)

- ½ teaspoon ground allspice (1/8 condiment)

Directions:

1. Toss all the ingredients for the broccoli bites in a mixing bowl, covering the broccoli florets on all sides.

2. Cook them in the preheated Air Fryer at 360 degrees for 13 to 15 minutes. In the meantime, mix all ingredients for the hot sauce.

3. Pause your Air Fryer, mix the broccoli with the prepared sauce and cook for a further 3 minutes. Bon appétit!

Nutrition:

- 70 Calories

- 4g Fat

- 2g Protein

47. Cheese Stuffed Mushrooms with Horseradish Sauce

Difficulty: Average

Preparation Time: 3 minutes

Cooking Time: 12 minutes

Servings: 5

Ingredients:

- 1/2 cup parmesan cheese, grated (1/4 healthy fat)

- 2 cloves garlic, pressed (1/4 condiment)

- 2 tablespoons fresh coriander, chopped (1/4 green)

- 1/3 teaspoon kosher salt (1/8 condiment)

- 1/2 teaspoon crushed red pepper flakes (1/8 condiment)

- 1 ½ tablespoons olive oil (1/4 condiment)

- 20 medium-sized mushrooms, cut off the stems (1 healthy fat)

- 1/2 cup Gorgonzola cheese, grated (1/2 healthy fat)

- 1/4 cup low-fat mayonnaise (1/4 healthy fat)

- 1 teaspoon prepared horseradish, well-drained (1/4 green)

- 1 tablespoon fresh parsley, finely chopped (1/4 green)

Directions:

1. Mix the parmesan cheese together with the garlic, coriander, salt, red pepper, and olive oil; mix to combine well.

2. Stuff the mushroom caps with the cheese filling. Top with grated Gorgonzola.

3. Place the mushrooms in the Air Fryer grill pan and slide them into the machine. Grill them at 380 degrees F for 8 to 12 minutes or until the stuffing is warmed through.

4. Meanwhile, prepare the horseradish sauce by mixing the mayonnaise, horseradish and parsley. Serve the horseradish sauce with the warm fried mushrooms. Enjoy!

Nutrition:

- 180 Calories

- 13.2g Fat

- 9g Protein

48. Broccoli with Herbs and Cheese

Difficulty: Average

Preparation Time: 8 minutes

Cooking Time: 17 minutes

Servings: 4

Ingredients:

- 1/3 cup grated yellow cheese (1/2 healthy fat)

- 1 large-sized head broccoli, stemmed and cut small florets (1 green)

- 2 1/2 tablespoons canola oil (1/8 condiment)

- 2 teaspoons dried rosemary (1/4 green)

- 2 teaspoons dried basil (1/4 green)

- Salt and ground black pepper to taste (1/8 condiment)

Directions:

1. Bring a medium pan filled with a lightly salted water to a boil. Then, boil the broccoli florets for about 3 minutes.

2. Then, drain the broccoli florets well; toss them with canola oil, rosemary, basil, salt and black pepper.

3. Set your oven to 390 degrees F; arrange the seasoned broccoli in the cooking basket; set the timer for 17 minutes. Toss the broccoli halfway through the cooking process.

4. Serve warm topped with grated cheese and enjoy!

Nutrition:

- 111 Calories

- 2.1g Fat

- 8.9g Protein

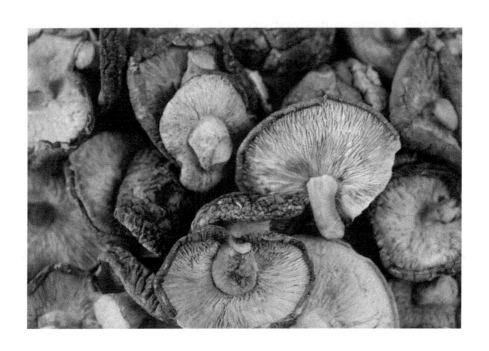

49. Family Favorite Stuffed Mushrooms

Difficulty: Easy

Preparation Time: 4 minutes

Cooking Time: 12 minutes

Servings: 2

Ingredients:

- 2 teaspoons cumin powder (1/4 condiment)

- 4 garlic cloves, peeled and minced (1/4 condiment)

- 18 medium-sized white mushrooms (2 healthy fats)

- Fine sea salt and freshly ground black pepper to taste (1/8 condiment)

- A pinch ground allspice (1/8 condiment)

- 2 tablespoons olive oil (1/4 condiment)

Directions:

1. First, clean the mushrooms; remove the middle stalks from the mushrooms to prepare the "shells."

2. Grab a mixing dish and thoroughly combine the remaining items. Fill the mushrooms with the prepared mixture.

3. Cook the mushrooms at 345 degrees F heat for 12 minutes. Enjoy!

Nutrition:

- 179 Calories

- 15g Fat

- 6g Protein

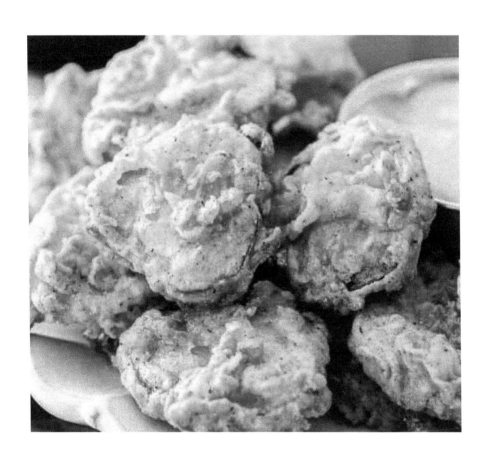

50. Famous Fried Pickles

Difficulty: Average

Preparation Time: 5 minutes

Cooking Time: 15 minutes

Servings: 6

Ingredients:

- 1/3 cup milk (1/2 healthy fat)
- 1 teaspoon garlic powder (1/8 condiment)
- 2 medium-sized eggs (1 healthy fat)
- 1 teaspoon fine sea salt (1/8 condiment)
- 1/3 teaspoon chili powder (1/4 condiment)
- 1/3 cup all-purpose flour (1/4 healthy fat)
- 1/2 teaspoon shallot powder (1/4 condiment)
- 2 jars sweet and sour pickle spears (1 healthy fat)

Directions:

1. Pat the pickle spears dry with a kitchen towel. Then take two mixing bowls.
2. Whisk the egg and milk in a bowl. In another bowl, combine all dry ingredients.

3. Firstly, dip the pickle spears into the dry mix; then coat each pickle with the egg/milk mixture; dredge them in the flour mixture again for additional coating.
4. Air fry battered pickles for 15 minutes at 385 degrees. Enjoy!

Nutrition:

- 58 Calories
- 2g Fat
- 3.2g Protein

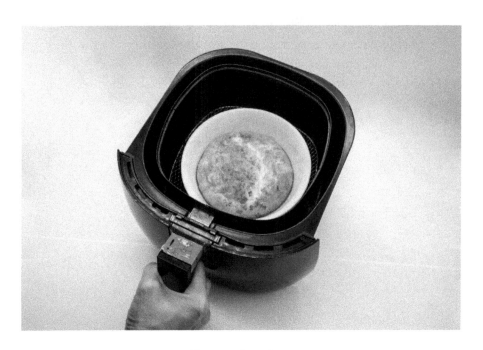

Conclusion

Cooking in an air fryer is an awesome way to cook food. Wheat flour breaded fish can be easily prepared in an air fryer, which results in crispy crusts and juicy insides. People on a diet should opt for air frying as it prepares food without frying and reduces the oil content by half. Air frying vegetable strips away the vegetable's excess water, which makes the vegetable delicious and tasty. Using this with your Lean and green diet is a great help. To make the diet much easier, you will be glad to know that lean and green food can be used along with air frying to make the diet much easier.

The Lean and Green diet is a diet which claims to be the healthiest and environmentally sustainable. It is also a diet which has good weight loss and muscle building properties.

The Lean and Green Diet is based on these principles: A predominantly plant-based diet with an emphasis on vegetables, fruits, whole grains and beans. A high level of physical activity (at least 30 minutes of aerobic exercise 3 times a week). Adherence to the nutritional recommendations from governmental food agencies (WCRF/AICR). Lastly, increased consumption of fish, poultry, whole-grains and low-fat dairy products (in the case of vegetarians). These 4 principles present a total package which promises to allow for the identification, identification and implementation of an effective lifestyle change. However, as with many other diets, the Lean and Green Diet has not been rigorously tested and thus it is often difficult to find scientific evidence for the diet's effectiveness.

However, there is scientific evidence for one of the principles: an environmental approach to food. For example, the use of recycled packaging at supermarkets could reduce a consumer's carbon footprint by 5-10%, according to the University of British Columbia. This is in comparison to the use of environmentally unfriendly packaging. There can also be environmental gains from reduced packaging from suppliers. For example, Anheuser-Busch uses windmills to reduce its energy usage by 25% and reduce the amount of carbon dioxide released into the atmosphere by 9%.

In relation to this, a key principle of Lean and Green is that it must be environmentally sustainable. It is often suggested that consumers take advantage of their purchasing power and bring about a change in the food system.

At this moment of your journey, you must recognize that you've overcome the hardest task, i.e., the first dreadful step towards health and wellbeing. Please remember that this alone is a commendable feat and whoever survives the first step can survive the rest and come out at the other side thinner, stronger, wiser, happier, and overall better.

Remember, the journey of a thousand miles still begins with just a single step indeed. So, stand tall, be confident, and just go ahead each day with your ideal vision of yourself in your mind, moving a bit closer to your goals every day.

The program has earned worldwide acclaim for its ability to deliver sustainable results without complicating people's meal program. It places very few food restrictions and inspires people to choose a healthier version of their daily food without compromising on taste and nutrition.